GLUTEN-FREE COOKBOOK FOR BEGINNERS

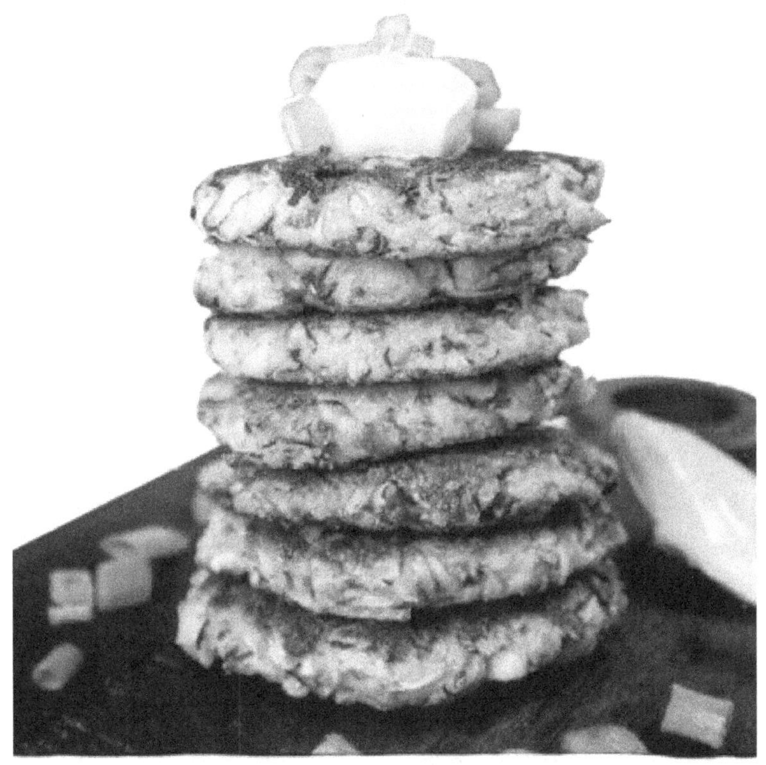

LORENE PEACHEY

DISCLAIMER

TO GAIN ACCESS TO MORE BOOK BY THE AUTHOR SCAN THE QR CODE

TABLE OF CONTENTS

INTRODUCTION

In the heart of culinary exploration, I find myself immersed in the delicious journey of crafting a gluten-free world—one where flavor knows no boundaries, and satisfaction comes without compromise. Allow me, Lorene Peachey, a seasoned nutritionist with 25 years of experience, to usher you into a realm where gluten-free living isn't just a lifestyle; it's an enchanting culinary adventure.

One day, as I navigated through the bustling aisles of a local grocery store, I encountered a remarkable woman named Stella, desperately seeking solace in the world of gluten-free cooking. Stella, with a vivacious spirit and a sparkle in her eyes, shared her culinary struggles with me, her frustrations evident as she recounted the countless times she had tried and failed with other cookbooks. A pang of empathy struck me as Stella poured her heart out, and I knew in that moment that my life's work had found a purpose—to transform not only Stella's kitchen but the kitchens of countless others yearning for a gluten-free sanctuary.

"Stella," I began with a warm smile, "I understand the challenges you've faced. It's disheartening when the recipes we try fall short of our expectations, isn't it?"

With a sigh, Stella nodded. "I've tried so many cookbooks, Lorene, but none seem to get it right. The frustration is real."

I empathetically reached out to Stella, assuring her that her struggles were not in vain. Little did she know that our conversation would unfold into a beautiful testament to the transformative power of gluten-free living.

As we delved into a dialogue, Stella shared the physical toll that gluten-rich diets had taken on her health. The bloating, the fatigue, the persistent digestive issues—

each symptom a poignant reminder of the consequences of consuming foods that her body could not tolerate.

I listened intently, my heart resonating with every word Stella uttered. In that moment, I realized that the true essence of gluten-free living went beyond the mere exclusion of gluten—it was about nourishing the body, embracing vitality, and indulging in a palette of flavors that brought joy to every bite.

"Stella, have you considered the profound impact of gluten-free living on your overall well-being?" I asked gently, guiding her towards the realization that gluten-free wasn't just a dietary restriction but a pathway to a healthier, more vibrant life.

As Stella embarked on the journey through my cookbook, named "Gluten-Free Cookbook for Beginners," a transformation unfolded. The once defeated gaze in Stella's eyes blossomed into a sparkle of newfound hope. Each recipe she explored became a testament to the power of mindful eating, and with each dish, she reclaimed control over her health and happiness.

"Can you believe it, Lorene? These recipes are a game-changer! My energy levels are up, and I feel lighter, both physically and emotionally," exclaimed Stella, her enthusiasm contagious.

Our conversation became a celebration of her culinary victories—of savoring the delectable almond flour banana muffins that danced on her taste buds, of relishing the zesty coconut flour banana bread that became a staple in her kitchen, and of reveling in the guilt-free pleasure of quinoa chocolate chip cookies that redefined her perception of what a cookie could be.

As I reflect on Stella's journey, I invite you, dear reader, to embark on your gluten-free odyssey. Picture a world where gluten-free isn't synonymous with limitation but rather an invitation to explore the rich tapestry of flavors that nature graciously provides.

Consider the benefits awaiting you as you step into the realm of gluten-free living. Feel the surge of energy that comes with nourishing your body with wholesome ingredients. Imagine the joy of enjoying meals that not only tantalize your taste buds but also contribute to your overall well-being.

Now, let's confront the pressing questions that linger in the air—questions that delve into the very core of our existence and the choices we make. What if your journey to gluten-free living could be a joyous exploration rather than a restrictive regimen? What if every meal could be a celebration of flavors, free from the constraints of gluten?

As a nutritionist, I must stress the dangers of consuming gluten-rich foods when one's body cannot tolerate them. The consequences extend beyond physical discomfort, impacting our energy levels, mental clarity, and overall vitality. The journey to gluten-free living isn't just a choice; it's a profound step towards reclaiming your health.

In this cookbook, meticulously curated over decades of research and experience, you'll discover not just recipes but a guide to a lifestyle that transcends the boundaries of dietary restrictions. Each page unfolds a narrative of healing, of joy, and of the endless possibilities that await when we choose to nourish ourselves with intention.

The advantages of having "Gluten-free Cookbook for Beginners" as your culinary companion are vast. With a friendly tone and clear instructions, even the most novice chef can whip up a feast that tantalizes the senses. The benefits extend beyond the kitchen, permeating every aspect of your life—from heightened energy levels to improved digestion, and from a clearer mind to a profound sense of well-being.

As you embark on this gluten-free journey, let the recipes within these pages be your compass, guiding you towards a world where gluten-free isn't a compromise; it's an elevation of your culinary experience. So, join me, Lorene Peachey, in this odyssey of flavors, and let the adventure unfold—one delicious recipe at a time. The gluten-free revolution begins with you, dear reader, and " Gluten-free Cookbook for Beginners " is your passport to a world of culinary bliss.

Contact the Author

Thank you for reading my book! I would love to hear from you, whether you have feedback, questions, or just want to share your thoughts. Your feedback means a lot to me and helps me improve as a writer.

Please don't hesitate to reach out to me through

lorenepeachey@gmail.com

I look forward to connecting with my readers and appreciate your support in this literary journey. Your thoughts and comments are valuable to me.

CHAPTER 1

UNDERSTANDING GLUTEN-FREE LIVING

Gluten-free living has gained significant attention in recent years, and many individuals are adopting a gluten-free diet for various reasons. Gluten is a protein found in wheat, barley, rye, and their derivatives. While some people follow a gluten-free lifestyle due to medical conditions like celiac disease or gluten sensitivity, others choose it for perceived health benefits. In this article, we will explore the key aspects of gluten-free living and the potential benefits associated with a gluten-free diet.

Celiac Disease and Gluten Sensitivity:

a. **Celiac Disease:** Celiac disease is an autoimmune disorder where the ingestion of gluten leads to damage in the small intestine. Individuals with celiac disease must strictly adhere to a gluten-free diet to manage symptoms and prevent long-term complications.

b. **Non-Celiac Gluten Sensitivity:** Some people experience symptoms similar to those of celiac disease without having the autoimmune response. This condition is known as non-celiac gluten sensitivity, and individuals with this sensitivity also benefit from avoiding gluten-containing foods.

Improved Digestive Health:

a. **Reduced Digestive Discomfort:** Adopting a gluten-free diet can alleviate digestive discomfort in individuals with gluten sensitivity or irritable bowel syndrome (IBS). Symptoms like bloating, gas, and abdominal pain often diminish with the elimination of gluten.

b. **Enhanced Nutrient Absorption:** For those with celiac disease, removing gluten from the diet allows the small intestine to heal, improving nutrient absorption. This is crucial for overall health, as malabsorption of nutrients can lead to deficiencies.

Increased Energy Levels:

a. **Balanced Blood Sugar Levels:** Some individuals report improved energy levels and better blood sugar control on a gluten-free diet. This may be attributed to the elimination of refined carbohydrates often found in gluten-containing foods.

b. **Reduced Fatigue:** Individuals with celiac disease may experience fatigue due to nutrient malabsorption. By following a gluten-free diet, nutrient absorption improves, potentially alleviating fatigue.

Potential Weight Management:

a. **Reduced Processed Foods Intake:** A gluten-free diet often involves avoiding many processed foods that contain gluten. By default, individuals may consume fewer processed and high-calorie foods, potentially contributing to weight management.

b. **Focus on Whole Foods:** Embracing a gluten-free lifestyle often encourages the consumption of whole, nutrient-dense foods such as fruits, vegetables, lean proteins, and gluten-free grains. This shift towards a healthier diet can aid in weight control.

CHAPTER 2

GETTING STARTED

Embarking on a gluten-free lifestyle involves more than just avoiding certain grains. It requires a fundamental understanding of gluten-containing foods, stocking up on gluten-free pantry essentials, and equipping your kitchen with the right tools to make gluten-free cooking enjoyable and stress-free. In this guide, we'll cover the essentials to help you get started on your gluten-free journey.

Identifying Gluten-Containing Foods:

Understanding which foods contain gluten is the first step towards a successful gluten-free lifestyle. Common sources of gluten include:

a. **Wheat:** Bread, pasta, cereals, and baked goods.

b. **Barley:** Malt, malt vinegar, and some alcoholic beverages.

c. **Rye:** Rye bread, some cereals, and certain alcoholic drinks.

d. **Oats:** While oats themselves are gluten-free, they are often contaminated during processing. Look for certified gluten-free oats.

e. **Hidden Sources:** Some processed foods, sauces, and condiments may contain hidden gluten. Always check labels for ingredients like wheat flour, modified starch, or malt extract.

Gluten-Free Pantry Essentials:

Stocking your pantry with gluten-free alternatives ensures you have the right ingredients at hand. Consider including:

a. **Gluten-Free Flours:** Almond flour, coconut flour, rice flour, and gluten-free flour blends can replace traditional wheat flour in various recipes.

b. **Whole Grains:** Quinoa, brown rice, millet, and gluten-free oats offer nutritious alternatives to gluten-containing grains.

c. **Legumes and Pulses:** Lentils, chickpeas, and beans are versatile, protein-rich options.

d. **Gluten-Free Pasta and Noodles:** Explore the variety of gluten-free pasta options made from rice, corn, or legumes.

e. **Gluten-Free Baking Essentials:** Baking powder, baking soda, and xanthan gum are crucial for gluten-free baking.

f. **Condiments and Sauces:** Opt for gluten-free soy sauce, tamari, and gluten-free versions of your favorite condiments.

g. **Snacks:** Keep a selection of gluten-free snacks such as nuts, seeds, popcorn, and gluten-free crackers.

Kitchen Tools for Gluten-Free Cooking:

Equipping your kitchen with the right tools makes gluten-free cooking efficient and enjoyable:

a. **Dedicated Gluten-Free Utensils:** To prevent cross-contamination, consider having separate cutting boards, knives, and utensils for gluten-free food preparation.

b. **Toaster Bags or Dedicated Toaster:** Avoid cross-contamination by using toaster bags or investing in a toaster exclusively for gluten-free bread.

c. **Food Processor or Blender:** Useful for creating gluten-free flours from grains or nuts.

d. **Mixing Bowls and Baking Pans:** Ensure you have an array of mixing bowls and baking pans for gluten-free baking.

e. **Labeling System:** Clearly label gluten-free items in your pantry and refrigerator to prevent mix-ups.

f. **Gluten-Free Cookbook:** Invest in a gluten-free cookbook or explore online resources for recipes and inspiration.

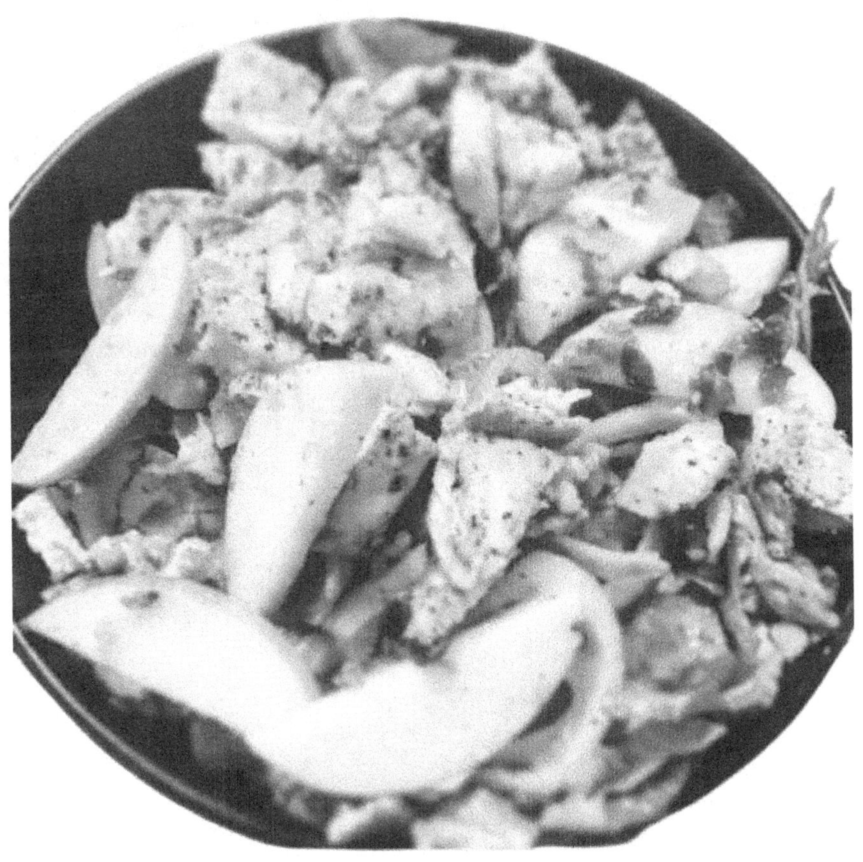

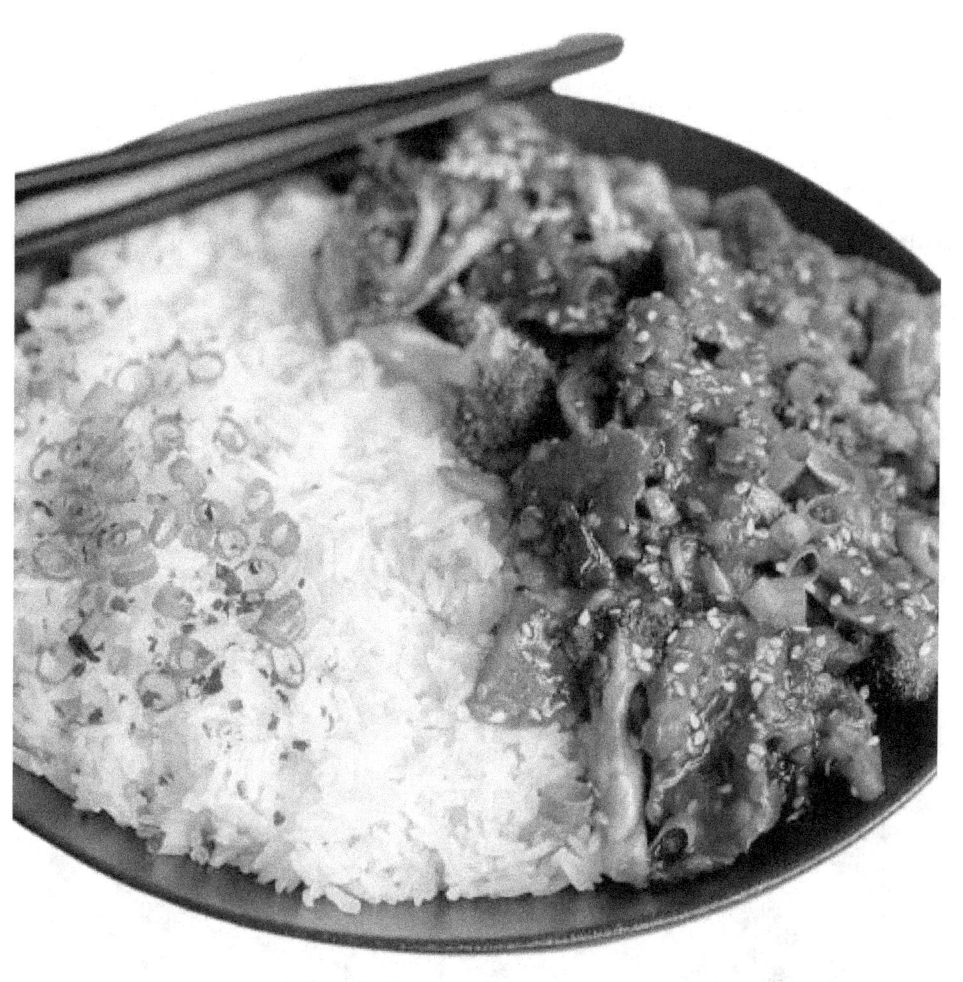

CHAPTER 3

BREAKFAST DELIGHTS

Quinoa Breakfast Bowl:

- **Cooking Time:** 15 minutes

- **Serving:** 2

- **Ingredients:**

    - 1 cup quinoa (cooked)

    - 1 cup almond milk

    - 1 banana (sliced)

    - 1/4 cup nuts (e.g., almonds, walnuts)

    - 1 tablespoon honey

- **Instructions:**

1. In a bowl, mix the cooked quinoa with almond milk until well combined.

2. Top the quinoa with sliced banana and your choice of nuts (e.g., almonds, walnuts).

3. Drizzle honey over the top for sweetness.

- **Nutritional Information:** 350 calories, 60g carbs, 10g protein, 8g fat, 6g fiber.

Begin your day with a protein-packed quinoa bowl loaded with fruits and nuts, providing sustained energy.

Gluten-Free Oat Pancakes:

- **Cooking Time:** 20 minutes

- **Serving:** 4

- **Ingredients:**

    - 2 cups gluten-free oats

    - 1 ripe banana

    - 1 cup almond milk

    - 1 teaspoon vanilla extract

- **Instructions:**

1.   In a blender, combine gluten-free oats, ripe banana, almond milk, and vanilla extract.

2.   Blend until smooth to create the pancake batter.

3.   Pour the batter onto a preheated griddle, cooking until both sides are golden brown.

- **Nutritional Information:** 200 calories, 35g carbs, 5g protein, 4g fat, 3g fiber.

Enjoy a guilt-free pancake breakfast using gluten-free oats for a wholesome and satisfying meal.

Greek Yogurt Parfait:

- **Preparation Time:** 10 minutes

- **Serving:** 1

- **Ingredients:**

    - 1 cup Greek yogurt

    - 1/2 cup gluten-free granola

    - 1/2 cup mixed berries

    - 1 tablespoon honey

- **Instructions:**

1.   In a glass or bowl, layer Greek yogurt with gluten-free granola and mixed berries.

2.   Drizzle honey over the top before serving.

- **Nutritional Information:** 250 calories, 30g carbs, 15g protein, 8g fat, 5g fiber.

Indulge in a protein-rich Greek yogurt parfait loaded with fresh berries and gluten-free granola for a delightful morning treat.

Spinach and Feta Omelette:

- **Cooking Time:** 10 minutes

- **Serving:** 1

- **Ingredients:**

    - 3 eggs

    - Handful of fresh spinach

    - 1/4 cup feta cheese (crumbled)

    - Salt and pepper to taste

- **Instructions:**

1. Whisk eggs in a bowl and pour into a heated pan.

2. Add fresh spinach, crumbled feta, salt, and pepper to the eggs.

3. Fold the omelette when set, ensuring even cooking.

- **Nutritional Information:** 280 calories, 4g carbs, 20g protein, 20g fat, 2g fiber.

Boost your morning with a protein-packed spinach and feta omelette, a quick and savory gluten-free breakfast option.

Banana Almond Chia Pudding:

- **Preparation Time:** 5 minutes (plus chilling time)

- **Serving:** 2

- **Ingredients:**

    - 2 ripe bananas

    - 1 cup almond milk

    - 1/4 cup chia seeds

    - 1 teaspoon vanilla extract

- **Instructions:**

1.   In a blender, combine ripe bananas, almond milk, and vanilla extract until smooth.

2.   Stir in chia seeds and refrigerate the mixture overnight.

- **Nutritional Information:** 220 calories, 30g carbs, 5g protein, 10g fat, 8g fiber.

Delight in a creamy banana almond chia pudding, a nutritious make-ahead option for a hassle-free morning.

Sweet Potato and Sausage Hash:

- **Cooking Time:** 25 minutes

- **Serving:** 2

- **Ingredients:**

    - 1 large sweet potato (diced)

    - 1/2 pound gluten-free sausage

    - 1 bell pepper (chopped)

    - 1 onion (diced)

- **Instructions:**

1. Cook gluten-free sausage in a pan until browned; set aside.

2. Sauté diced sweet potato, chopped bell pepper, and diced onion in the same pan until vegetables are tender.

3. Mix in the cooked sausage before serving.

- **Nutritional Information:** 320 calories, 25g carbs, 15g protein, 18g fat, 5g fiber.

Experience a savory sweet potato and sausage hash, a hearty and flavorful gluten-free breakfast to kickstart your day.

Avocado and Tomato Breakfast Toast:

- **Preparation Time:** 10 minutes

- **Serving:** 2

- **Ingredients:**

  - 4 slices gluten-free bread

  - 1 ripe avocado

  - 1 tomato (sliced)

  - Salt, pepper, and red pepper flakes to taste

- **Instructions:**

1. Toast gluten-free bread slices until golden brown.

2. Spread mashed avocado evenly on each slice.

3. Top with tomato slices and season with salt, pepper, and red pepper flakes.

- **Nutritional Information:** 280 calories, 30g carbs, 5g protein, 16g fat, 6g fiber.

Elevate your breakfast with a nutrient-packed avocado and tomato toast, a simple yet satisfying gluten-free option.

Blueberry Almond Smoothie Bowl:

- **Preparation Time:** 10 minutes

- **Serving:** 1

- **Ingredients:**

    - 1 cup frozen blueberries

    - 1/2 banana

    - 1/2 cup almond milk

    - 2 tablespoons almond butter

- **Instructions:**

1. Blend frozen blueberries, banana, almond milk, and almond butter until smooth.

2. Pour the smoothie into a bowl and top with sliced almonds for added crunch.

- **Nutritional Information:** 280 calories, 35g carbs, 8g protein, 15g fat, 7g fiber.

Start your day with a refreshing blueberry almond smoothie bowl, packed with antioxidants and healthy fats.

Rice Cake with Smoked Salmon and Cream Cheese:

- **Preparation Time:** 15 minutes

- **Serving:** 2

- **Ingredients:**

    - 4 gluten-free rice cakes

    - 4 ounces smoked salmon

    - 1/2 cup cream cheese

    - Fresh dill for garnish

- **Instructions:**

1. Spread cream cheese evenly on each gluten-free rice cake.

2. Top with slices of smoked salmon and garnish with fresh dill.

- **Nutritional Information:** 260 calories, 25g carbs, 15g protein, 12g fat, 2g fiber.

Indulge in a sophisticated rice cake topped with smoked salmon and cream cheese for a protein-rich gluten-free breakfast.

Mango Coconut Chia Seed Pudding:

- **Preparation Time:** 10 minutes (plus chilling time)

- **Serving:** 2

- **Ingredients:**

    - 1 ripe mango (diced)

    - 1 cup coconut milk

    - 1/4 cup chia seeds

    - 1 teaspoon honey (optional)

- **Instructions:**

1. In a bowl, mix diced ripe mango with coconut milk.

2. Stir in chia seeds and let the mixture chill in the refrigerator for a few hours or overnight.

3. Optionally, drizzle honey on top before serving.

- **Nutritional Information:** 240 calories, 30g carbs, 4g protein, 12g fat, 8g fiber.

Savor the tropical flavors of mango and coconut in this chia seed pudding—a delightful and nutritious gluten-free breakfast option.

CHAPTER 4

APPETIZERS AND SNACKS

Guacamole with Veggie Sticks

- **Preparation Time:** 10 minutes

- **Serving:** 4

- **Ingredients:**

    - 3 ripe avocados

    - 1 tomato (diced)

    - 1/2 red onion (finely chopped)

    - 1 lime (juiced)

    - Salt and pepper to taste

    - Assorted veggie sticks (carrots, cucumbers, bell peppers)

- **Instructions:**

1. Mash avocados in a bowl and mix in diced tomatoes, chopped red onion, lime juice, salt, and pepper.

2. Serve with a variety of veggie sticks.

- **Nutritional Information:** 150 calories, 12g carbs, 2g protein, 11g fat, 7g fiber.

Indulge in a classic guacamole paired with colorful veggie sticks—a healthy and satisfying gluten-free snack.

Caprese Skewers:

- **Preparation Time:** 15 minutes

- **Serving:** 6

- **Ingredients:**

  - Cherry tomatoes

  - Fresh mozzarella balls

  - Fresh basil leaves

  - Balsamic glaze

  - Olive oil

  - Salt and pepper to taste

- **Instructions:**

1. Thread cherry tomatoes, mozzarella balls, and basil leaves onto skewers.

2. Drizzle with balsamic glaze and olive oil; season with salt and pepper.

- **Nutritional Information:** 120 calories, 5g carbs, 6g protein, 9g fat, 1g fiber.

Enjoy the vibrant flavors of a classic Caprese salad in convenient skewer form—a delightful gluten-free appetizer.

Hummus with Gluten-Free Pita Chips:

- **Preparation Time:** 15 minutes

- **Serving:** 8

- **Ingredients:**

    - 2 cans chickpeas (drained)

    - 1/4 cup tahini

    - 2 cloves garlic

    - 1/4 cup olive oil

    - 2 tablespoons lemon juice

    - Gluten-free pita chips (for dipping)

- **Instructions:**

1. Blend chickpeas, tahini, garlic, olive oil, and lemon juice until smooth.

2. Serve with gluten-free pita chips.

- **Nutritional Information:** 180 calories, 20g carbs, 6g protein, 10g fat, 4g fiber.

Whip up a creamy hummus paired with gluten-free pita chips—a classic and versatile gluten-free snack.

Quinoa Stuffed Mushrooms:

- **Preparation Time:** 30 minutes

- **Serving:** 12

- **Ingredients:**

    - 1 cup quinoa (cooked)

    - 24 button mushrooms

    - 1/2 cup feta cheese (crumbled)

    - 1/4 cup chopped fresh parsley

    - 2 tablespoons olive oil

    - Salt and pepper to taste

- **Instructions:**

1. Remove stems from mushrooms and set aside.

2. In a bowl, mix cooked quinoa, feta cheese, chopped parsley, olive oil, salt, and pepper.

3. Stuff mushrooms with the quinoa mixture.

4. Bake until mushrooms are tender.

- **Nutritional Information:** 120 calories, 15g carbs, 4g protein, 6g fat, 2g fiber.

Elevate your appetizer game with quinoa-stuffed mushrooms—a gluten-free, flavorful twist on a classic dish.

Zucchini Fritters:

- **Preparation Time:** 20 minutes

- **Serving:** 4

- **Ingredients:**

  - 2 medium zucchinis (grated)

  - 1/4 cup gluten-free breadcrumbs

  - 1/4 cup grated Parmesan cheese

  - 1 egg

  - 2 tablespoons chopped fresh dill

  - Salt and pepper to taste

- **Instructions:**

1. Squeeze excess water from grated zucchini.

2. In a bowl, combine zucchini, breadcrumbs, Parmesan, egg, dill, salt, and pepper.

3. Form mixture into fritters and cook until golden brown.

- **Nutritional Information:** 110 calories, 10g carbs, 6g protein, 5g fat, 2g fiber.

Savor the crispiness of gluten-free zucchini fritters—a delightful and healthy snack or appetizer.

Devilled Eggs with Smoked Paprika:

- **Preparation Time:** 15 minutes

- **Serving:** 12

- **Ingredients:**

    - 6 hard-boiled eggs

    - 1/4 cup mayonnaise

    - 1 teaspoon Dijon mustard

    - Smoked paprika for garnish

    - Salt and pepper to taste

- **Instructions:**

1. Halve hard-boiled eggs and remove yolks.

2. Mix yolks with mayonnaise, Dijon mustard, salt, and pepper.

3. Spoon the mixture back into egg whites and sprinkle with smoked paprika.

- **Nutritional Information:** 90 calories, 1g carbs, 6g protein, 7g fat, 0g fiber.

Classic deviled eggs with a touch of smoked paprika—an elegant and protein-packed gluten-free appetizer.

Stuffed Bell Peppers with Quinoa and Black Beans:

- **Preparation Time:** 40 minutes

- **Serving:** 6

- **Ingredients:**

    - 3 bell peppers (halved)

    - 1 cup quinoa (cooked)

    - 1 can black beans (drained and rinsed)

    - 1 cup corn kernels

    - 1 cup salsa

    - 1 cup shredded cheddar cheese

- **Instructions:**

1. Preheat the oven and halve bell peppers.

2. In a bowl, mix cooked quinoa, black beans, corn, and salsa.

3. Stuff bell peppers with the quinoa mixture and top with shredded cheddar.

4. Bake until peppers are tender.

- **Nutritional Information:** 280 calories, 40g carbs, 12g protein, 8g fat, 8g fiber.

Enjoy a nutritious and flavorful gluten-free option with stuffed bell peppers filled with quinoa, black beans, and cheese.

Smoky Roasted Chickpeas:

- **Preparation Time:** 30 minutes

- **Serving:** 4

- **Ingredients:**

    - 2 cans chickpeas (drained and patted dry)

    - 2 tablespoons olive oil

    - 1 teaspoon smoked paprika

    - 1/2 teaspoon cumin

    - Salt and cayenne pepper to taste

- **Instructions:**

1. Toss chickpeas in olive oil, smoked paprika, cumin, salt, and cayenne.

2. Roast until chickpeas are crispy.

- **Nutritional Information:** 160 calories, 20g carbs, 7g protein, 7g fat, 5g fiber.

Satisfy your crunchy cravings with smoky roasted chickpeas—a protein-packed gluten-free snack.

Salmon Cucumber Bites:

- **Preparation Time:** 15 minutes

- **Serving:** 4

- **Ingredients:**

    - Cucumber slices

    - Smoked salmon

    - Cream cheese

    - Fresh dill for garnish

- **Instructions:**

1. Top cucumber slices with cream cheese.

2. Add a slice of smoked salmon on top.

3. Garnish with fresh dill.

- **Nutritional Information:** 120 calories, 3g carbs, 10g protein, 8g fat, 1g fiber.

Delight in the freshness of salmon cucumber bites —a simple and elegant gluten-free appetizer.

Buffalo Cauliflower Bites:

- **Preparation Time:** 25 minutes

- **Serving:** 4

- **Ingredients:**

    - 1 head cauliflower (cut into florets)

    - 1/2 cup gluten-free flour

    - 1/2 cup buffalo sauce

    - 2 tablespoons melted butter

    - 1 teaspoon garlic powder

    - Ranch dressing (for dipping)

- **Instructions:**

1. Toss cauliflower florets in gluten-free flour.

2. Bake until golden brown.

3. In a bowl, mix buffalo sauce, melted butter, and garlic powder.

4. Coat baked cauliflower in the buffalo sauce mixture.

- **Nutritional Information:** 150 calories, 20g carbs, 4g protein, 7g fat, 4g fiber.

Experience the bold flavors of buffalo cauliflower bites—a tasty gluten-free alternative to traditional wings.

<h1 style="text-align:center">CHAPTER 5</h1>

<h1 style="text-align:center">SATISFYING SOUPS</h1>

Roasted Tomato Basil Soup:

- **Cooking Time:** 45 minutes

- **Serving:** 6

- **Ingredients:**

    - 6 large tomatoes (quartered)

    - 1 onion (chopped)

    - 3 cloves garlic (minced)

    - 2 tablespoons olive oil

    - 4 cups vegetable broth

    - 1 cup fresh basil leaves

- **Instructions:**

1. Toss tomatoes, onion, and garlic with olive oil; roast until caramelized.

2. Blend roasted vegetables with vegetable broth and fresh basil.

3. Simmer the mixture until heated through.

- **Nutritional Information:** 120 calories, 15g carbs, 3g protein, 7g fat, 4g fiber.

Indulge in the rich flavors of a homemade roasted tomato basil soup—a comforting gluten-free option perfect for chilly days.

Butternut Squash and Apple Soup:

- **Cooking Time:** 40 minutes

- **Serving:** 4

- **Ingredients:**

    - 1 medium butternut squash (peeled and cubed)

    - 2 apples (peeled and chopped)

    - 1 onion (chopped)

    - 4 cups vegetable broth

    - 1 teaspoon cinnamon

    - Salt and pepper to taste

- **Instructions:**

1. Sauté onion until softened; add butternut squash and apples.

2. Pour in vegetable broth, season with cinnamon, salt, and pepper.

3. Simmer until squash is tender, then blend until smooth.

- **Nutritional Information:** 150 calories, 35g carbs, 2g protein, 1g fat, 5g fiber.

Experience the sweetness of butternut squash and apples in a velvety gluten-free soup—a fall-inspired delight.

Chicken and Vegetable Quinoa Soup:

- **Cooking Time:** 30 minutes

- **Serving:** 6

- **Ingredients:**

    - 1 cup quinoa (rinsed)

    - 1 pound chicken breast (cooked and shredded)

    - 1 onion (chopped)

    - 2 carrots (sliced)

    - 2 celery stalks (chopped)

    - 6 cups chicken broth

- **Instructions:**

1. Cook quinoa separately according to package instructions.

2. In a pot, sauté onion, carrots, and celery.

3. Add shredded chicken, cooked quinoa, and chicken broth; simmer until vegetables are tender.

- **Nutritional Information:** 220 calories, 20g carbs, 25g protein, 4g fat, 3g fiber.

Enjoy a hearty and protein-packed chicken and vegetable quinoa soup—a fulfilling gluten-free meal for any occasion.

Lentil and Kale Soup:

- **Cooking Time:** 35 minutes

- **Serving:** 5

- **Ingredients:**

    - 1 cup green lentils (rinsed)

    - 1 onion (chopped)

    - 3 carrots (sliced)

    - 2 cloves garlic (minced)

    - 4 cups vegetable broth

    - 2 cups chopped kale

- **Instructions:**

1. Sauté onion and garlic; add carrots, lentils, and vegetable broth.

2. Simmer until lentils are tender, then stir in chopped kale.

3. Continue simmering until kale is wilted.

- **Nutritional Information:** 180 calories, 30g carbs, 12g protein, 1g fat, 10g fiber.

Delight in the nourishing goodness of lentil and kale soup—a gluten-free option bursting with flavors and nutrients.

Creamy Broccoli and Cheddar Soup:

- **Cooking Time:** 25 minutes

- **Serving:** 4

- **Ingredients:**

    - 4 cups broccoli florets

    - 1 onion (chopped)

    - 2 cups vegetable broth

    - 1 cup shredded cheddar cheese

    - 1 cup milk (dairy or plant-based)

- **Instructions:**

1. Sauté onion until softened; add broccoli and vegetable broth.

2. Simmer until broccoli is tender, then blend until smooth.

3. Stir in cheddar cheese and milk until melted and creamy.

- **Nutritional Information:** 250 calories, 20g carbs, 12g protein, 15g fat, 5g fiber.

Satisfy your cravings with a velvety, gluten-free broccoli and cheddar soup—a comforting classic for any day.

Shrimp and Corn Chowder:

- **Cooking Time:** 35 minutes

- **Serving:** 5

- **Ingredients:**

    - 1 pound shrimp (peeled and deveined)

    - 2 cups corn kernels

    - 1 onion (chopped)

    - 2 potatoes (peeled and diced)

    - 4 cups chicken broth

    - 1 cup milk (dairy or plant-based)

- **Instructions:**

1. Sauté shrimp and onion; add diced potatoes, corn, and chicken broth.

2. Simmer until potatoes are tender, then stir in milk.

3. Cook until shrimp are pink and fully cooked.

- **Nutritional Information:** 280 calories, 30g carbs, 20g protein, 8g fat, 3g fiber.

Savor the flavors of the sea with a delightful shrimp and corn chowder—a gluten-free soup that's both hearty and satisfying.

Thai Coconut Curry Soup:

- **Cooking Time:** 40 minutes

- **Serving:** 4

- **Ingredients:**

  - 1 pound chicken thighs (boneless and skinless, sliced)

  - 1 can coconut milk

  - 2 tablespoons red curry paste

  - 1 bell pepper (sliced)

  - 1 cup sliced mushrooms

  - 2 tablespoons fish sauce

  - 1 tablespoon lime juice

- **Instructions:**

1. Cook chicken in a pot; add coconut milk and red curry paste.

2. Stir in sliced bell pepper, mushrooms, fish sauce, and lime juice.

3. Simmer until vegetables are tender and flavors meld.

- **Nutritional Information:** 320 calories, 8g carbs, 20g protein, 24g fat, 2g fiber.

Transport your taste buds with a Thai coconut curry soup—a gluten-free dish that combines bold flavors with comfort.

Potato Leek Soup:

- **Cooking Time:** 30 minutes

- **Serving:** 6

- **Ingredients:**

    - 4 potatoes (peeled and diced)

    - 2 leeks (cleaned and sliced)

    - 4 cups vegetable broth

    - 1 cup milk (dairy or plant-based)

    - 2 tablespoons olive oil

- **Instructions:**

1. Sauté leeks in olive oil until softened; add diced potatoes and vegetable broth.

2. Simmer until potatoes are tender, then blend until smooth.

3. Stir in milk until well combined.

- **Nutritional Information:** 200 calories, 30g carbs, 5g protein, 8g fat, 3g fiber.

Warm up with a creamy and flavorful potato leek soup—a gluten-free classic that's both simple and satisfying.

Mexican Black Bean Soup:

- **Cooking Time:** 25 minutes

- **Serving:** 4

- **Ingredients:**

    - 2 cans black beans (drained and rinsed)

    - 1 onion (chopped)

    - 1 bell pepper (chopped)

    - 2 cloves garlic (minced)

    - 4 cups vegetable broth

    - 1 teaspoon cumin

- **Instructions:**

1. Sauté onion, bell pepper, and garlic until softened; add black beans, vegetable broth, and cumin.

2. Simmer until flavors meld and beans are tender.

- **Nutritional Information:** 180 calories, 30g carbs, 10g protein, 1g fat, 8g fiber.

Embark on a flavor journey with a Mexican black bean soup—a gluten-free dish that's hearty, healthy, and delicious.

Spinach and White Bean Soup:

- **Cooking Time:** 30 minutes

- **Serving:** 5

- **Ingredients:**

    - 1 onion (chopped)

    - 2 carrots (sliced)

    - 2 celery stalks (chopped)

    - 3 cloves garlic (minced)

    - 4 cups vegetable broth

    - 1 can white beans (drained and rinsed)

    - 2 cups fresh spinach leaves

- **Instructions:**

1.   Sauté onion, carrots, celery, and garlic until softened; add vegetable broth and bring to a simmer.

2.   Stir in white beans and fresh spinach until wilted.

- **Nutritional Information:** 150 calories, 30g carbs, 8g protein, 1g fat, 6g fiber.

Nourish your body with a gluten-free spinach and white bean soup—a comforting and wholesome option for any day.

CHAPTER 6

SALADS FOR EVERY SEASON

Spring Strawberry Spinach Salad

- **Preparation Time:** 15 minutes

- **Serving:** 4

- **Ingredients:**

    - 6 cups fresh baby spinach

    - 1 cup sliced strawberries

    - 1/2 cup crumbled feta cheese

    - 1/4 cup sliced almonds

    - Balsamic vinaigrette dressing

- **Instructions:**

1. Toss baby spinach with sliced strawberries, feta cheese, and sliced almonds.

2. Drizzle with balsamic vinaigrette before serving.

- **Nutritional Information:** 180 calories, 15g carbs, 8g protein, 12g fat, 4g fiber.

Embrace the freshness of spring with a vibrant strawberry spinach salad—a gluten-free option bursting with color and flavor.

Summer Caprese Salad:

- **Preparation Time:** 10 minutes

- **Serving:** 4

- **Ingredients:**

    - 4 large tomatoes (sliced)

    - 1 pound fresh mozzarella (sliced)

    - Fresh basil leaves

    - Balsamic glaze

    - Olive oil

    - Salt and pepper to taste

- **Instructions:**

1. Arrange tomato and mozzarella slices on a platter.

2. Tuck fresh basil leaves between slices, drizzle with balsamic glaze and olive oil.

3. Season with salt and pepper.

- **Nutritional Information:** 250 calories, 8g carbs, 14g protein, 18g fat, 2g fiber.

Celebrate the flavors of summer with a classic Caprese salad—a gluten-free dish that's simple, elegant, and delicious.

Autumn Harvest Quinoa Salad:

- **Preparation Time:** 20 minutes

- **Serving:** 6

- **Ingredients:**

    - 2 cups cooked quinoa

    - 1 cup diced butternut squash (roasted)

    - 1 cup dried cranberries

    - 1/2 cup chopped pecans

    - 1/4 cup feta cheese (optional)

    - Maple Dijon dressing

- **Instructions:**

1. Mix cooked quinoa with roasted butternut squash, cranberries, pecans, and feta.

2. Drizzle with maple Dijon dressing and toss gently.

- **Nutritional Information:** 280 calories, 45g carbs, 6g protein, 10g fat, 5g fiber.

Enjoy the flavors of autumn with a hearty harvest quinoa salad—a gluten-free option featuring seasonal ingredients.

Winter Citrus Kale Salad:

- **Preparation Time:** 15 minutes

- **Serving:** 4

- **Ingredients:**

  - 4 cups chopped kale

  - 2 oranges (peeled and segmented)

  - 1/2 cup pomegranate arils

  - 1/4 cup chopped almonds

  - Feta cheese crumbles

  - Citrus vinaigrette dressing

- **Instructions:**

1. Massage chopped kale with citrus vinaigrette until tender.

2. Toss with orange segments, pomegranate arils, chopped almonds, and feta cheese.

- **Nutritional Information:** 220 calories, 30g carbs, 8g protein, 10g fat, 6g fiber.

Brighten up winter days with a refreshing citrus kale salad—a gluten-free dish that's both nutritious and satisfying.

Grilled Chicken Caesar Salad:

- **Preparation Time:** 25 minutes

- **Serving:** 2

- **Ingredients:**

  - 2 boneless, skinless chicken breasts

  - Romaine lettuce hearts

  - Gluten-free croutons

  - Shaved Parmesan cheese

  - Caesar dressing

- **Instructions:**

1. Grill chicken breasts until fully cooked; slice.

2. Arrange romaine lettuce on plates, top with grilled chicken, gluten-free croutons, and shaved Parmesan.

3. Drizzle with Caesar dressing.

- **Nutritional Information:** 320 calories, 15g carbs, 35g protein, 15g fat, 5g fiber.

Savor a classic with a gluten-free twist—grilled chicken Caesar salad, a hearty and satisfying option for any time of year.

Mediterranean Quinoa Salad:

- **Preparation Time:** 20 minutes

- **Serving:** 4

- **Ingredients:**

    - 2 cups cooked quinoa

    - Cherry tomatoes (halved)

    - Cucumber (diced)

    - Kalamata olives (sliced)

    - Red onion (finely chopped)

    - Feta cheese crumbles

    - Greek vinaigrette dressing

- **Instructions:**

1.	Combine cooked quinoa with cherry tomatoes, cucumber, olives, red onion, and feta.

2.	Toss with Greek vinaigrette dressing.

- **Nutritional Information:** 240 calories, 30g carbs, 8g protein, 10g fat, 5g fiber.

Take your taste buds on a trip to the Mediterranean with a gluten-free quinoa salad—fresh, flavorful, and packed with nutrients.

Asian Noodle Salad with Shrimp:

- **Preparation Time:** 30 minutes

- **Serving:** 4

- **Ingredients:**

  - Rice noodles (cooked)

  - Shrimp (peeled and deveined)

  - Shredded cabbage

  - Carrots (julienned)

  - Edamame

  - Sesame seeds

  - Soy ginger dressing

- **Instructions:**

1. Cook rice noodles and shrimp; let them cool.

2. Toss noodles, shrimp, shredded cabbage, julienned carrots, and edamame.

3. Drizzle with soy ginger dressing and sprinkle sesame seeds.

- **Nutritional Information:** 280 calories, 35g carbs, 20g protein, 8g fat, 5g fiber.

Experience the vibrant flavors of Asia with an Asian noodle salad featuring shrimp—a gluten-free dish that's both tasty and satisfying.

Southwest Black Bean and Corn Salad:

- **Preparation Time:** 15 minutes

- **Serving:** 6

- **Ingredients:**

    - 1 can black beans (drained and rinsed)

    - 1 cup corn kernels (fresh or thawed)

    - Cherry tomatoes (halved)

    - Avocado (diced)

    - Red onion (finely chopped)

    - Fresh cilantro (chopped)

    - Lime vinaigrette dressing

- **Instructions:**

1.   Combine black beans, corn, cherry tomatoes, avocado, red onion, and cilantro.

2.   Toss with lime vinaigrette dressing.

- **Nutritional Information:** 220 calories, 35g carbs, 8g protein, 8g fat, 7g fiber.

Spice up your salad game with a flavorful Southwest black bean and corn salad—a gluten-free dish that's perfect for a quick, nutritious meal.

Greek Chickpea Salad:

- **Preparation Time:** 20 minutes

- **Serving:** 4

- **Ingredients:**

  - 2 cans chickpeas (drained and rinsed)

  - Cucumber (diced)

  - Cherry tomatoes (halved)

  - Red onion (finely chopped)

  - Feta cheese crumbles

  - Kalamata olives (sliced)

  - Greek dressing

- **Instructions:**

1. Mix chickpeas with cucumber, cherry tomatoes, red onion, feta, and olives.

2. Toss with Greek dressing.

- **Nutritional Information:** 260 calories, 30g carbs, 10g protein, 12g fat, 8g fiber.

Enjoy the vibrant flavors of the Mediterranean with a gluten-free Greek chickpea salad—fresh, satisfying, and loaded with goodness.

Apple Walnut Chicken Salad:

- **Preparation Time:** 25 minutes

- **Serving:** 4

- **Ingredients:**

  - Grilled chicken breast (sliced)

  - Mixed salad greens

  - Apple (thinly sliced)

  - Walnuts (chopped)

  - Goat cheese crumbles

  - Apple cider vinaigrette dressing

- **Instructions:**

1. Arrange mixed salad greens on plates; top with grilled chicken, apple slices, walnuts, and goat cheese.

2. Drizzle with apple cider vinaigrette dressing.

- **Nutritional Information:** 280 calories, 20g carbs, 25g protein, 15g fat, 5g fiber.

Elevate your salad experience with an apple walnut chicken salad—a gluten-free option that combines sweet and savory elements for a delightful meal.

CHAPTER 7

MAIN COURSE MARVELS

Baked Lemon Garlic Herb Salmon:

- **Cooking Time:** 20 minutes

- **Serving:** 4

- **Ingredients:**

    - 4 salmon fillets

    - 2 tablespoons olive oil

    - 2 cloves garlic (minced)

    - Lemon zest and juice

    - Fresh herbs (such as parsley or dill)

    - Salt and pepper to taste

- **Instructions:**

1. Preheat oven; place salmon on a baking sheet.

2. Mix olive oil, minced garlic, lemon zest, lemon juice, and fresh herbs; pour over salmon.

3. Bake until salmon is cooked through.

- **Nutritional Information:** 300 calories, 0g carbs, 30g protein, 20g fat, 0g fiber.

Elevate your dinner with the freshness of baked lemon garlic herb salmon—a gluten-free main course that's both flavorful and nutritious.

Quinoa Stuffed Bell Peppers:

- **Cooking Time:** 40 minutes

- **Serving:** 6

- **Ingredients:**

    - 1 cup quinoa (cooked)

    - 6 bell peppers (halved)

    - Ground turkey or beef

    - Onion (chopped)

    - Tomato sauce

    - Shredded cheese

- **Instructions:**

1. Cook quinoa and brown ground meat with chopped onion.

2. Mix quinoa and meat; stuff bell peppers and top with tomato sauce and cheese.

3. Bake until peppers are tender.

- **Nutritional Information:** 280 calories, 30g carbs, 20g protein, 10g fat, 6g fiber.

Enjoy a wholesome gluten-free meal with quinoa-stuffed bell peppers—a delicious and customizable dish for any occasion.

Chicken and Vegetable Stir-Fry:

- **Cooking Time:** 25 minutes

- **Serving:** 4

- **Ingredients:**

    - 1 pound chicken breast (sliced)

    - Assorted vegetables (broccoli, bell peppers, snap peas)

    - Gluten-free soy sauce

    - Garlic and ginger (minced)

    - Sesame oil

    - Rice or gluten-free noodles

- **Instructions:**

1.   Sauté chicken until cooked; set aside.

2.   Stir-fry assorted vegetables with minced garlic and ginger.

3.   Add cooked chicken, gluten-free soy sauce, and sesame oil; serve over rice or noodles.

- **Nutritional Information:** 320 calories, 25g carbs, 30g protein, 12g fat, 5g fiber.

Whip up a quick and flavorful gluten-free chicken and vegetable stir-fry—a perfect balance of protein and veggies for a satisfying meal.

Eggplant Parmesan:

- **Cooking Time:** 45 minutes

- **Serving:** 5

- **Ingredients:**

    - 2 large eggplants (sliced)

    - Gluten-free breadcrumbs

    - Marinara sauce

    - Mozzarella and Parmesan cheese

    - Fresh basil

- **Instructions:**

1. Coat eggplant slices in gluten-free breadcrumbs; bake until golden.

2. Layer baked eggplant with marinara sauce, mozzarella, Parmesan, and fresh basil.

3. Bake until bubbly and golden.

- **Nutritional Information:** 250 calories, 25g carbs, 10g protein, 12g fat, 8g fiber.

Indulge in the Italian flavors of gluten-free eggplant Parmesan—a comforting and hearty main course for any day.

Shrimp and Vegetable Skewers:

- **Cooking Time:** 15 minutes

- **Serving:** 4

- **Ingredients:**

    - 1 pound large shrimp (peeled and deveined)

    - Assorted vegetables (bell peppers, cherry tomatoes, zucchini)

    - Olive oil

    - Garlic powder, paprika, salt, and pepper

    - Lemon wedges

- **Instructions:**

1. Thread shrimp and vegetables onto skewers.

2. Brush with olive oil, sprinkle with garlic powder, paprika, salt, and pepper.

3. Grill until shrimp are pink and veggies are tender.

- **Nutritional Information:** 180 calories, 10g carbs, 25g protein, 8g fat, 3g fiber.

Savor the simplicity of grilled shrimp and vegetable skewers—a gluten-free, low-calorie option for a quick and tasty meal.

Turkey and Sweet Potato Hash:

- **Cooking Time:** 30 minutes

- **Serving:** 4

- **Ingredients:**

    - 1 pound ground turkey

    - Sweet potatoes (diced)

    - Onion (chopped)

    - Bell peppers (chopped)

    - Garlic (minced)

    - Smoked paprika, cumin, salt, and pepper

- **Instructions:**

1. Brown ground turkey; set aside.

2. Sauté sweet potatoes, onion, bell peppers, and garlic until tender.

3. Mix in cooked turkey and season with smoked paprika, cumin, salt, and pepper.

- **Nutritional Information:** 280 calories, 25g carbs, 25g protein, 10g fat, 4g fiber.

Fuel your day with a protein-packed and gluten-free turkey and sweet potato hash—a hearty and flavorful choice for breakfast or dinner.

Baked Chicken Parmesan:

- **Cooking Time:** 40 minutes

- **Serving:** 4

- **Ingredients:**

    - 4 boneless, skinless chicken breasts

    - Gluten-free breadcrumbs

    - Marinara sauce

    - Mozzarella and Parmesan cheese

    - Fresh basil

- **Instructions:**

1. Coat chicken breasts in gluten-free breadcrumbs; bake until golden.

2. Top with marinara sauce, mozzarella, Parmesan, and fresh basil.

3. Bake until cheese is melted and bubbly.

- **Nutritional Information:** 320 calories, 20g carbs, 30g protein, 15g fat, 2g fiber.

Enjoy the classic flavors of chicken Parmesan in a gluten-free version—a delicious and satisfying main course for any night.

Spaghetti Squash with Pesto and Cherry Tomatoes:

- **Cooking Time:** 45 minutes

- **Serving:** 4

- **Ingredients:**

    - 1 spaghetti squash

    - Pesto sauce

    - Cherry tomatoes (halved)

    - Pine nuts

    - Fresh basil

- **Instructions:**

1. Roast spaghetti squash; scrape into strands.

2. Toss squash with pesto, cherry tomatoes, pine nuts, and fresh basil.

3. Serve warm.

- **Nutritional Information:** 220 calories, 30g carbs, 4g protein, 12g fat, 5g fiber.

Experience a light and flavorful meal with spaghetti squash topped with pesto and cherry tomatoes—a gluten-free alternative to traditional pasta.

Beef and Broccoli Stir-Fry:

- **Cooking Time:** 20 minutes

- **Serving:** 4

- **Ingredients:**

    - 1 pound beef sirloin (sliced)

    - Broccoli florets

    - Gluten-free soy sauce

    - Sesame oil

    - Garlic and ginger (minced)

    - Rice or gluten-free noodles

- **Instructions:**

1. Sauté sliced beef until browned; set aside.

2. Stir-fry broccoli with minced garlic and ginger.

3. Add cooked beef, gluten-free soy sauce, and sesame oil; serve over rice or noodles.

- **Nutritional Information:** 340 calories, 20g carbs, 30g protein, 15g fat, 4g fiber.

Enjoy the savory combination of beef and broccoli in a gluten-free stir-fry—a quick and satisfying main course for busy evenings.

Lentil and Vegetable Curry:

- **Cooking Time:** 35 minutes

- **Serving:** 6

- **Ingredients:**

    - 1 cup green lentils (rinsed)

    - Assorted vegetables (carrots, peas, bell peppers)

    - Coconut milk

    - Curry powder, cumin, coriander, turmeric

    - Garlic and ginger (minced)

    - Basmati rice

- **Instructions:**

1. Cook lentils separately; set aside.

2. Sauté assorted vegetables with minced garlic and ginger.

3. Mix in cooked lentils, coconut milk, curry powder, cumin, coriander, and turmeric; serve over basmati rice.

- **Nutritional Information:** 280 calories, 40g carbs, 15g protein, 8g fat, 8g fiber.

Delight your taste buds with a flavorful lentil and vegetable curry—a gluten-free and plant-based main course perfect for a satisfying dinner.

CHAPTER 8
28 DAY MEAL PLAN

Week 1:

Day 1:

- **Breakfast:** Almond Flour Banana Muffins
- **Lunch:** Quinoa Salad with Grilled Chicken
- **Dinner:** Baked Lemon Garlic Salmon with Roasted Vegetables
- **Snack:** Chia Seed Pudding with Berries

Day 2:

- **Breakfast:** Oatmeal Raisin Cookies
- **Lunch:** Lentil and Vegetable Curry
- **Dinner:** Gluten-Free Zucchini Bread with a side salad
- **Snack:** Fresh Fruit

Day 3:

- **Breakfast:** Coconut Flour Banana Bread Slices
- **Lunch:** Sweet Potato Brownies (Gluten-Free and Vegan)
- **Dinner:** Beef and Broccoli Stir-Fry with Quinoa
- **Snack:** Sliced Cucumber with Hummus

Day 4:

- **Breakfast:** Flourless Chocolate Avocado Brownies

- **Lunch:** Gluten-Free Lemon Blueberry Muffins with Greek Yogurt

- **Dinner:** Chicken and Vegetable Stir-Fry with Buckwheat Noodles

- **Snack:** Quinoa Chocolate Chip Cookies

Day 5:

- **Breakfast:** Buckwheat Banana Pancakes with Maple Syrup

- **Lunch:** Gluten-Free Zucchini Bread with Turkey and Avocado Sandwich

- **Dinner:** Spaghetti Squash with Pesto and Cherry Tomatoes

- **Snack:** Mixed Nuts

Day 6:

- **Breakfast:** Quinoa Chocolate Chip Cookies

- **Lunch:** Lentil and Vegetable Curry

- **Dinner:** Grilled Shrimp Skewers with Quinoa

- **Snack:** Apple Slices with Almond Butter

Day 7:

- **Breakfast:** Chia Seed Pudding with Berries

- **Lunch:** Gluten-Free Lemon Blueberry Muffins with Cottage Cheese

- **Dinner:** Baked Chicken with Roasted Vegetables

- **Snack:** Fresh Fruit Salad

Week 2:

Day 8:

- **Breakfast:** Almond Flour Banana Muffins

- **Lunch:** Quinoa Salad with Grilled Chicken

- **Dinner:** Baked Lemon Garlic Salmon with Roasted Vegetables

- **Snack:** Chia Seed Pudding with Berries

Day 9:

- **Breakfast:** Oatmeal Raisin Cookies

- **Lunch:** Lentil and Vegetable Curry

- **Dinner:** Gluten-Free Zucchini Bread with a side salad

- **Snack:** Fresh Fruit

Day 10:

- **Breakfast:** Coconut Flour Banana Bread Slices

- **Lunch:** Sweet Potato Brownies (Gluten-Free and Vegan)

- **Dinner:** Beef and Broccoli Stir-Fry with Quinoa

- **Snack:** Sliced Cucumber with Hummus

Day 11:

- **Breakfast:** Flourless Chocolate Avocado Brownies

- **Lunch:** Gluten-Free Lemon Blueberry Muffins with Greek Yogurt

- **Dinner:** Chicken and Vegetable Stir-Fry with Buckwheat Noodles

- **Snack:** Quinoa Chocolate Chip Cookies

Day 12:

- **Breakfast:** Buckwheat Banana Pancakes with Maple Syrup

- **Lunch:** Gluten-Free Zucchini Bread with Turkey and Avocado Sandwich

- **Dinner:** Spaghetti Squash with Pesto and Cherry Tomatoes

- **Snack:** Mixed Nuts

Day 13:

- **Breakfast:** Quinoa Chocolate Chip Cookies

- **Lunch:** Lentil and Vegetable Curry

- **Dinner:** Grilled Shrimp Skewers with Quinoa

- **Snack:** Apple Slices with Almond Butter

Day 14:

- **Breakfast:** Chia Seed Pudding with Berries

- **Lunch:** Gluten-Free Lemon Blueberry Muffins with Cottage Cheese

- **Dinner:** Baked Chicken with Roasted Vegetables

- **Snack:** Fresh Fruit Salad

Week 3:

Day 15:

- **Breakfast:** Almond Flour Banana Muffins

- **Lunch:** Quinoa Salad with Grilled Chicken

- **Dinner:** Baked Lemon Garlic Salmon with Roasted Vegetables

- **Snack:** Chia Seed Pudding with Berries

Day 16:

- **Breakfast:** Oatmeal Raisin Cookies

- **Lunch:** Lentil and Vegetable Curry

- **Dinner:** Gluten-Free Zucchini Bread with a side salad

- **Snack:** Fresh Fruit

Day 17:

- **Breakfast:** Coconut Flour Banana Bread Slices

- **Lunch:** Sweet Potato Brownies (Gluten-Free and Vegan)

- **Dinner:** Beef and Broccoli Stir-Fry with Quinoa

- **Snack:** Sliced Cucumber with Hummus

Day 18:

- **Breakfast:** Flourless Chocolate Avocado Brownies

- **Lunch:** Gluten-Free Lemon Blueberry Muffins with Greek Yogurt

- **Dinner:** Chicken and Vegetable Stir-Fry with Buckwheat Noodles

- **Snack:** Quinoa Chocolate Chip Cookies

Day 19:

- **Breakfast:** Buckwheat Banana Pancakes with Maple Syrup

- **Lunch:** Gluten-Free Zucchini Bread with Turkey and Avocado Sandwich

- **Dinner:** Spaghetti Squash with Pesto and Cherry Tomatoes

- **Snack:** Mixed Nuts

Day 20:

- **Breakfast:** Quinoa Chocolate Chip Cookies

- **Lunch:** Lentil and Vegetable Curry

- **Dinner:** Grilled Shrimp Skewers with Quinoa

- **Snack:** Apple Slices with Almond Butter

Day 21:

- **Breakfast:** Chia Seed Pudding with Berries

- **Lunch:** Gluten-Free Lemon Blueberry Muffins with Cottage Cheese

- **Dinner:** Baked Chicken with Roasted Vegetables

- **Snack:** Fresh Fruit Salad

Week 4:

Day 22:

- **Breakfast:** Almond Flour Banana Muffins

- **Lunch:** Quinoa Salad with Grilled Chicken

- **Dinner:** Baked Lemon Garlic Salmon with Roasted Vegetables

- **Snack:** Chia Seed Pudding with Berries

Day 23:

- **Breakfast:** Oatmeal Raisin Cookies

- **Lunch:** Lentil and Vegetable Curry

- **Dinner:** Gluten-Free Zucchini Bread with a side salad

- **Snack:** Fresh Fruit

Day 24:

- **Breakfast:** Coconut Flour Banana Bread Slices

- **Lunch:** Sweet Potato Brownies (Gluten-Free and Vegan)

- **Dinner:** Beef and Broccoli Stir-Fry with Quinoa

- **Snack:** Sliced Cucumber with Hummus

Day 25:

- **Breakfast:** Flourless Chocolate Avocado Brownies

- **Lunch:** Gluten-Free Lemon Blueberry Muffins with Greek Yogurt

- **Dinner:** Chicken and Vegetable Stir-Fry with Buckwheat Noodles

- **Snack:** Quinoa Chocolate Chip Cookies

Day 26:

- **Breakfast:** Buckwheat Banana Pancakes with Maple Syrup

- **Lunch:** Gluten-Free Zucchini Bread with Turkey and Avocado Sandwich

- **Dinner:** Spaghetti Squash with Pesto and Cherry Tomatoes

- **Snack:** Mixed Nuts

Day 27:

- **Breakfast:** Quinoa Chocolate Chip Cookies

- **Lunch:** Lentil and Vegetable Curry

- **Dinner:** Grilled Shrimp Skewers with Quinoa

- **Snack:** Apple Slices with Almond Butter

Day 28:

- **Breakfast:** Chia Seed Pudding with Berries

- **Lunch:** Gluten-Free Lemon Blueberry Muffins with Cottage Cheese

- **Dinner:** Baked Chicken with Roasted Vegetables

- **Snack:** Fresh Fruit Salad

CONCLUSION

As we come to the delightful conclusion of our gluten-free odyssey, I am filled with gratitude for the opportunity to share this culinary adventure with you. Through "Gluten-free Cookbook for Beginners," we've explored the vast landscapes of gluten-free living, transforming not just meals but lifestyles. I hope the pages of this cookbook have ignited a spark of inspiration within you, encouraging a shift towards a healthier, more flavourful existence.

As you embark on your gluten-free journey, remember that each recipe is a stepping stone towards a revitalized you. The benefits are not only found in the wholesome ingredients but in the joy of creating, savouring, and sharing meals that nourish the body and soul. With every bite, you are reclaiming your health and celebrating the abundance of Flavors that nature provides.

Your feedback is invaluable on this culinary expedition. I encourage you to share your experiences, triumphs, and even the delightful challenges you may encounter. Your insights will not only enhance this cookbook but contribute to a community of individuals embracing a gluten-free lifestyle. Your journey is unique, and your voice adds to the vibrant tapestry of stories woven through these recipes.'\

Feel free to reach out with questions, suggestions, or to share your favorite creations. The gluten-free community is one of support, encouragement, and shared passion for wholesome living. Together, we can turn every meal into a celebration, every recipe into a story, and every bite into a moment of joy.

May " Gluten-free Cookbook for Beginners " be a cherished companion in your kitchen, guiding you towards a future of health, happiness, and culinary delight. From my kitchen to yours, thank you for joining me on this flavourful odyssey

BONUS CHAPTER

10 HEALTHY GLUTEN-FREE BAKING RECIPES

Almond Flour Banana Muffins

- **Cooking Time:** 25 minutes

- **Serving:** 12 muffins

- **Ingredients:**

    - 2 cups almond flour

    - 3 ripe bananas (mashed)

    - 3 eggs

    - 1/4 cup honey or maple syrup

    - 1 teaspoon baking soda

    - 1/2 teaspoon vanilla extract

- **Instructions:**

1.   Preheat the oven to 350°F (175°C) and line a muffin tin with paper liners.

2.   In a large mixing bowl, combine almond flour, mashed bananas, eggs, honey or maple syrup, baking soda, and vanilla extract.

3.   Mix the ingredients until well combined and a batter forms.

4.   Spoon the batter into the muffin cups, filling each about 2/3 full.

5.   Bake in the preheated oven for 20-25 minutes or until a toothpick inserted into the center of a muffin comes out clean.

6.   Allow the muffins to cool in the tin for 5 minutes before transferring them to a wire rack to cool completely.

- **Nutritional Information:** 150 calories, 15g carbs, 5g protein, 9g fat, 3g fiber.

Indulge in guilt-free almond flour banana muffins—a gluten-free treat that's both delicious and wholesome.

Oatmeal Raisin Cookies (Gluten-Free):

- **Cooking Time:** 15 minutes

- **Serving:** 18 cookies

- **Ingredients:**

  - 2 cups gluten-free oats

  - 1 cup almond flour

  - 1/2 cup coconut oil (melted)

  - 1/2 cup maple syrup

  - 2 eggs

  - 1 teaspoon ground cinnamon

  - 1/2 cup raisins

- **Instructions:**

1. Preheat the oven to 350°F (175°C) and line a baking sheet with parchment paper.

2. In a large bowl, combine gluten-free oats, almond flour, melted coconut oil, maple syrup, eggs, ground cinnamon, and raisins.

3. Mix the ingredients until well combined and a cookie dough forms.

4. Scoop tablespoon-sized portions of dough and place them onto the prepared baking sheet.

5. Flatten each cookie slightly with the back of a spoon.

6.   Bake in the preheated oven for 12-15 minutes or until the edges are golden brown.

7.   Allow the cookies to cool on the baking sheet for 5 minutes before transferring them to a wire rack to cool completely.

- **Nutritional Information:** 120 calories, 15g carbs, 2g protein, 6g fat, 2g fiber.

Enjoy the chewy goodness of gluten-free oatmeal raisin cookies—a wholesome twist on a classic favorite.

Flourless Chocolate Avocado Brownies:

- **Cooking Time:** 30 minutes

- **Serving:** 16 brownies

- **Ingredients:**

  - 2 ripe avocados (mashed)

  - 1/2 cup cocoa powder

  - 1/2 cup honey or maple syrup

  - 2 eggs

  - 1 teaspoon vanilla extract

  - 1/2 teaspoon baking soda

  - Pinch of salt

- **Instructions:**

1. Preheat the oven to 350°F (175°C) and grease a square baking pan.

2. In a bowl, combine mashed avocados, cocoa powder, honey or maple syrup, eggs, vanilla extract, baking soda, and a pinch of salt.

3. Mix until smooth and well combined.

4. Pour the batter into the prepared baking pan.

5. Bake for 25-30 minutes or until a toothpick inserted into the center comes out with a few moist crumbs.

6. Allow the brownies to cool in the pan before cutting into squares.

- **Nutritional Information:** 130 calories, 15g carbs, 2g protein, 8g fat, 3g fiber.

Satisfy your chocolate cravings with flourless chocolate avocado brownies—a gluten-free, fudgy delight.

Gluten-Free Lemon Blueberry Muffins:

- **Cooking Time:** 20 minutes

- **Serving:** 12 muffins

- **Ingredients:**

    - 2 cups gluten-free flour

    - 1/2 cup coconut oil (melted)

    - 1/2 cup honey or maple syrup

    - 2 eggs

    - 1 cup fresh blueberries

    - Zest and juice of 1 lemon

    - 1 teaspoon baking powder

- **Instructions:**

1. Preheat the oven to 375°F (190°C) and line a muffin tin with paper liners.

2. In a large bowl, mix gluten-free flour, melted coconut oil, honey or maple syrup, eggs, fresh blueberries, lemon zest, lemon juice, and baking powder.

3. Stir until the ingredients are well combined.

4. Spoon the batter into the muffin cups, filling each about 2/3 full.

5. Bake for 15-20 minutes or until a toothpick inserted into the center comes out clean.

6. Allow the muffins to cool in the tin for 5 minutes before transferring them to a wire rack.

- **Nutritional Information:** 160 calories, 20g carbs, 2g protein, 8g fat, 2g
  fiber.

Brighten your day with gluten-free lemon blueberry muffins—a burst of citrus and berries in every bite.

Coconut Flour Banana Bread:

- **Cooking Time:** 50 minutes

- **Serving:** 10 slices

- **Ingredients:**

    - 1 cup coconut flour

    - 4 ripe bananas (mashed)

    - 4 eggs

    - 1/4 cup coconut oil (melted)

    - 1/4 cup honey or maple syrup

    - 1 teaspoon baking soda

    - 1 teaspoon vanilla extract

- **Instructions:**

1. Preheat the oven to 350°F (175°C) and grease a loaf pan.

2. In a large bowl, combine coconut flour, mashed bananas, eggs, melted coconut oil, honey or maple syrup, baking soda, and vanilla extract.

3. Mix until smooth and well incorporated.

4. Pour the batter into the prepared loaf pan.

5. Bake for 45-50 minutes or until a toothpick inserted into the center comes out clean.

6. Allow the banana bread to cool in the pan before slicing.

- **Nutritional Information:** 180 calories, 25g carbs, 4g protein, 8g fat, 5g fiber.

Enjoy a slice of moist and flavorful coconut flour banana bread—a gluten-free twist on a classic favorite.

Quinoa Chocolate Chip Cookies:

- **Cooking Time:** 18 minutes

- **Serving:** 24 cookies

- **Ingredients:**

  - 1 cup cooked quinoa (cooled)

  - 1 cup gluten-free flour

  - 1/2 cup coconut oil (melted)

  - 1/2 cup coconut sugar

  - 1 egg

  - 1 teaspoon vanilla extract

  - 1/2 teaspoon baking soda

  - 1/4 teaspoon salt

  - 1 cup gluten-free chocolate chips

- **Instructions:**

1. Preheat the oven to 375°F (190°C) and line a baking sheet with parchment paper.

2. In a bowl, combine cooked quinoa, gluten-free flour, melted coconut oil, coconut sugar, egg, vanilla extract, baking soda, and salt.

3. Mix until well combined, then fold in the gluten-free chocolate chips.

4. Drop spoonfuls of dough onto the prepared baking sheet.

5. Bake for 15-18 minutes or until the edges are golden brown.

6.   Allow the cookies to cool on the baking sheet for 5 minutes before transferring them to a wire rack.

- **Nutritional Information:** 110 calories, 15g carbs, 2g protein, 6g fat, 1g fiber.

Savor the goodness of quinoa chocolate chip cookies—a gluten-free, protein-packed treat for cookie lovers.

Sweet Potato Brownies (Gluten-Free and Vegan):

- **Cooking Time:** 35 minutes

- **Serving:** 16 brownies

- **Ingredients:**

  - 1 cup sweet potato puree

  - 1/2 cup almond butter

  - 1/4 cup maple syrup

  - 1/4 cup cocoa powder

  - 1 teaspoon vanilla extract

  - 1/2 teaspoon baking powder

  - 1/4 teaspoon sea salt

  - 1/2 cup dairy-free chocolate chips

- **Instructions:**

1.   Preheat the oven to 350°F (175°C) and line a square baking pan with parchment paper.

2.   In a bowl, combine sweet potato puree, almond butter, maple syrup, cocoa powder, vanilla extract, baking powder, and sea salt.

3.   Mix until smooth, then fold in the dairy-free chocolate chips.

4.   Pour the batter into the prepared baking pan.

5.   Bake for 25-30 minutes or until a toothpick inserted into the center comes out with a few moist crumbs.

6.   Allow the brownies to cool in the pan before cutting into squares.

- **Nutritional Information:** 120 calories, 15g carbs, 2g protein, 6g fat, 2g fiber.

Indulge in decadent sweet potato brownies—a gluten-free and vegan option for a guilt-free chocolate treat.

Gluten-Free Zucchini Bread:

- **Cooking Time:** 50 minutes

- **Serving:** 12 slices

- **Ingredients:**

  - 2 cups shredded zucchini

  - 2 cups gluten-free flour

  - 1/2 cup coconut oil (melted)

  - 1/2 cup honey or maple syrup

  - 3 eggs

  - 1 teaspoon baking powder

  - 1/2 teaspoon baking soda

  - 1 teaspoon cinnamon

- **Instructions:**

1. Preheat the oven to 350°F (175°C) and grease a loaf pan.

2. In a large bowl, combine shredded zucchini, gluten-free flour, melted coconut oil, honey or maple syrup, eggs, baking powder, baking soda, and cinnamon.

3. Mix until well combined.

4. Pour the batter into the prepared loaf pan.

5. Bake for 45-50 minutes or until a toothpick inserted into the center comes out clean.

6.   Allow the zucchini bread to cool in the pan before slicing.

- **Nutritional Information:** 150 calories, 20g carbs, 3g protein, 7g fat, 2g fiber.

Enjoy a moist and flavorful slice of gluten-free zucchini bread—a delicious way to sneak in some veggies.

Chia Seed Pudding with Berries:

- **Prep Time:** 5 minutes (plus chilling time)

- **Serving:** 4

- **Ingredients:**

    - 1/2 cup chia seeds

    - 2 cups almond milk

    - 1 teaspoon vanilla extract

    - 2 tablespoons maple syrup

    - Fresh berries for topping

- **Instructions:**

1. In a bowl, whisk together chia seeds, almond milk, vanilla extract, and maple syrup.

2. Cover and refrigerate for at least 2 hours or overnight until the mixture thickens.

3. Stir well before serving and top with fresh berries.

- **Nutritional Information:** 120 calories, 15g carbs, 4g protein, 6g fat, 8g fiber.

Delight in a healthy and gluten-free chia seed pudding with berries—a simple and nutritious dessert or breakfast option.

Buckwheat Banana Pancakes:

- **Cooking Time:** 15 minutes

- **Serving:** 8 pancakes

- **Ingredients:**

    - 1 cup buckwheat flour

    - 2 ripe bananas (mashed)

    - 2 eggs

    - 1 cup almond milk

    - 1 teaspoon baking powder

    - 1/2 teaspoon cinnamon

    - Coconut oil for cooking

- **Instructions:**

1. In a bowl, combine buckwheat flour, mashed bananas, eggs, almond milk, baking powder, and cinnamon.

2. Mix until the batter is smooth.

3. Heat a skillet over medium heat and add coconut oil.

4. Spoon the batter onto the skillet to form pancakes.

5. Cook until bubbles form on the surface, then flip and cook the other side.

6. Serve warm with your favorite toppings.

- **Nutritional Information:** 140 calories, 20g carbs, 5g protein, 5g fat, 3g fiber.

Start your day with a stack of fluffy buckwheat banana pancakes—a gluten-free and wholesome breakfast option.

WEEKLY PLANNER

MONDAY	TUESDAY

WEDNESDAY	THURSDAY

FRIDAY	SATUREDAY

SUNDAY	NOTE

WEEKLY PLANNER

MONDAY	TUESDAY

WEDNESDAY	THURSDAY

FRIDAY	SATUREDAY

SUNDAY	NOTE

WEEKLY PLANNER

MONDAY

TUESDAY

WEDNESDAY

THURSDAY

FRIDAY

SATUREDAY

SUNDAY

NOTE

WEEKLY PLANNER

MONDAY	TUESDAY

WEDNESDAY	THURSDAY

FRIDAY	SATUREDAY

SUNDAY	NOTE

WEEKLY PLANNER

MONDAY	TUESDAY

WEDNESDAY	THURSDAY

FRIDAY	SATUREDAY

SUNDAY	NOTE

WEEKLY PLANNER

MONDAY	TUESDAY

WEDNESDAY	THURSDAY

FRIDAY	SATUREDAY

SUNDAY	NOTE

WEEKLY PLANNER

MONDAY	TUESDAY

WEDNESDAY	THURSDAY

FRIDAY	SATUREDAY

SUNDAY	NOTE

WEEKLY PLANNER

MONDAY	TUESDAY

WEDNESDAY	THURSDAY

FRIDAY	SATUREDAY

SUNDAY	NOTE

WEEKLY PLANNER

MONDAY

TUESDAY

WEDNESDAY

THURSDAY

FRIDAY

SATUREDAY

SUNDAY

NOTE